DON'T QUIT!

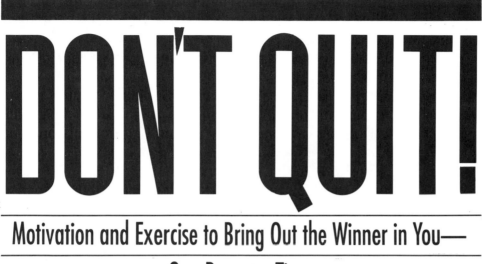

DON'T QUIT!

Motivation and Exercise to Bring Out the Winner in You—

One Day at a Time

JAKE STEINFELD

WARNER BOOKS

A Time Warner Company

Warner Books, Inc., 1271 Avenue of the Americas, New York, NY 10020

W A Time Warner Company

Printed in the United States of America
First Printing: May 1993
10 9 8 7 6 5 4 3 2 1

Library of Congress Cataloging-in-Publication Data

Steinfeld, Jake.
    Don't quit : motivation and exercise to bring out the winner in you, one day at a time / Jake Steinfeld.
        p.   cm.
    ISBN 0-446-39485-8
    1. Exercise.   2. Motivation (Psychology)   3. Self-management (Psychology)   I. Title.
GV481.S723   1993
613.7'1—dc20   92—31250
                                                                                                           CIP

Cover photo by Herman Estevez
Cover design by Diane Luger
Book design by Giorgetta Bell McRee

To my beautiful wife Tracey
and my precious new daughter Morgan.
I am the luckiest guy in the world.

CONTENTS

ACKNOWLEDGMENTS

Howard Polskin—the man who took my words and put them on these pages.

Steven "Wiels" Spielberg—to my "Big Brother." I couldn't have learned the business from a better person.

John Landis—for launching my acting career.

Tim Robertson—there are very few people in this world who say they're going to do something and then do it. Tim Robertson is that kind of guy.

Phil Scotti—the only other man who has Body by Jake running through his veins.

Michele Anselmo—for single-handedly keeping the Body by Jake machine running like a finely-tuned Rolls Royce.

Jamie Raab—the best editor an author can ask for.

INTRODUCTION

This is a book about bringing out the winner in you...one day at a time. It's about shaping up—and not being down. I want to push you to be successful, optimistic, organized, and happy. I want to pump you up so BIG in your mind that you'll approach every day in the most positive frame of mind.

This is a book about change. Changing your life ONE DAY AT A TIME. That's why I've divided the book into three key sections: the MORNING PUMP, the MIDDAY KICKER, and the EVENING PEP TALK. It will help you break down your major goals into a series of smaller, easier-to-reach targets. It will get you accustomed to thinking positively and productively in each part of the day, *one day at a time.*

I've also included exercise and nutrition chapters. This is not just a book about expanding your mind. It's about shrinking your waistline, and increasing your energy. If you feel great about your body, it's easier to feel great about yourself.

For more than a decade, I've trained some of the biggest stars and executives in Hollywood. The more weight they lost, the heavier my reputation became. I became successful not just because I knew

1

how to get my clients in shape. I also worked on their minds. That was the key. I considered myself more than a trainer. I was a motivator. And the more I worked with my clients, the more motivated I became to become the best person I could be.

Their success rubbed off on me. I personally saw how they went about their work. I listened. I learned.

And now I want to tell you what I learned in the past thirteen years.

About success.
About getting into shape.
About having a positive attitude.
About organization.
About being the best person you can be.

1

MY STORY
A True Tale of Inspiration, Motivation, and Perspiration

My goal in this book is to motivate you to believe in yourself and become the most productive, positive person you can be.

That's a tall order.

But it works. I have proof.

Me.

The story of my success shows how I—an average, regular guy—became the premier trainer to the stars, a TV personality, and a successful businessman. Not bad for someone who avoided school-work, was out of shape, and dreaded speaking in public. How I did it is partly a tale of luck and partly being in the right place at the right time. But mostly it's about perseverance and having a positive attitude.

IN THE BEGINNING...

I was a fat kid.

Really.

Born in Brooklyn. Raised on Long Island.

I loved sports. I hated studying. I had a stutter. I was not on anybody's "Most likely to succeed" list. Far from it.

But I was lucky that I came from a great family. I have younger twin brothers and a younger sister. My parents are terrific people. They always believed in me. They offered only positive suggestions. I felt virtually immune to failure.

Until eighth grade....

In eighth grade I went out for the basketball team. I figured all I had to do was show up and I'd be the starting forward for the Baldwin Junior High School basketball team.

I went through a week of tryouts. And I'll never forget, at the end of that week, going to the gym bulletin board on Friday afternoon where they posted the names of the guys who made the team.

I walked over knowing I was on the team.

Just about everything in my life until that moment had gone my way. I walked over to that wall slapping people five because I couldn't conceive that I wasn't going to make that team. I reached the concrete wall. I looked at the names.

And my name wasn't on the list!

I pulled the paper off the wall to look behind it. I thought someone was playing a joke on me. It finally hit me that I didn't make the team. This was the first time I was judged publicly...AND I LOST!

That was devastating to me.

But I distinctly remember saying to myself, "This is not going to be like this for long."

To cheer me up, a friend gave me a poem called "Don't Quit." I've lived by that poem since that day. The poem helped get me through the sense of failure and get me back on the road to success.

My dad immediately put up a basketball hoop in the back yard. I'd shoot baskets while my brothers would rebound. I played basketball every waking hour. The next year in ninth grade, I made the team. In tenth grade, I ended up as the captain.

That was my first experience with a major defeat. And I wouldn't accept it. It made me not just a better basketball player but a better person. I took that failure and turned it into a success. That became a blueprint for the rest of my life.

HOW I GOT PHYSICAL

My dad bought me a set of weights in the summer after eighth grade. He put them in the backyard. He called me outside and said we should lift some weights. I was a pudgy, overweight kid at the time. Twinkies in hand, I said, "No thank you."

A week later I brought them into my room. I picked up the weights and put Frank Sinatra's "My Way" on my stereo. Don't ask me why I ever listened to this record. At the end of the album there were ten seconds of wild applause for Frank Sinatra. But I hooked into this applause. I kept listening to the ten seconds of wild applause. And I'd do my bicep curls to the screaming audience.

I formed a mental picture of myself, Jake Steinfeld, doing bicep curls in front of 50,000 screaming fans in Madison Square Garden. I knew then I was destined for something in the public spotlight.

Fortunately, my body responded to the weights. One day, I was a husky kid. Within a month I had trimmed down. And my fat was being replaced with muscle. Friends started noticing my new body. They'd say, "Ooh, Jake Steinfeld. Big arms, pal."

As I was working out, I was gaining confidence in myself. When you're in good shape, people look at you in a different way. I learned that fast.

There was a definite correlation among how I looked, how I felt about myself, and how the outside world perceived me.

At this time, I also had a terrible stutter. Getting up and talking in front of a class was my biggest fear.

Can you imagine that? Me. A guy who today gets up before an

audience of a thousand and, without notes or a script, talks for an hour. A guy who appears daily on national television.

When we'd have to read out loud in class, I could barely handle it. I could tell a story or a joke in front of my friends without stuttering. But I had this block about reading in front of the class. I would have preferred to swim with sharks than read out loud in school.

I never had any type of formal therapy to overcome my stutter. I was fortunate that my parents were understanding and supportive in the way they handled my stutter. But by far the biggest factor in overcoming my stutter was my body building. As my muscles became bigger, my stutter became smaller.

Cut to eleventh grade. At the time I was lifting weights almost all the time. And when I wasn't lifting I was reading the body-building magazines. So I entered my first body-building contest. My family drove me to Delaware for the competition. There was one thing about them: they were (and still are) 100 percent behind me in everything I did. They always showed they were behind me.

The contestants drew numbers for the order of posing. My plan was to watch several guys to see how they posed. They would serve as my model. They'd give me an idea what to do on the stage. I didn't even know how to put oil on my body.

I was very scared. But I instinctively did then what I do now. I just threw myself into the situation wholeheartedly. Instead of wading into the shallow end, I jumped into the deep end. This contest was one of the first times I exhibited this trait, which is so much a part of me now. Inside I was shaking, but I had to learn how to take those butterflies and turn them into eagles.

I looked at the other twenty-three guys in the competition and thought to myself, "Man, these are real body builders! What am I doing here?"

When it came time to draw a number, I got number one. I was the first guy on the stage to pose.

Did I fold? No way. I had watched several body-building contests over the years and, in a near panic, I forced myself to recall how those body builders posed and acted on stage. Subconsciously, I had been preparing for this moment for the past two years with my complete immersion in the sport. Everything I read and learned came back to me in one dazzling rush.

I must have done something right because I came in fifth place and took home a trophy. I went home a winner.

No, it wasn't just me. It was all of us...my mother, father, sister, and brothers. My team. We went home winners. I couldn't have done it without them. I was mentally prepared because of my family's support. That fifth-place finish taught me how to plunge headfirst into a new situation and succeed. And it also taught me the value of support from family and friends.

CALIFORNIA DREAMING

I went to Cortland State College in Cortland, New York. My body may have been in the snow of upstate New York, but my mind was already in the warm California sun. That's where I knew I was going to pursue my goal to become the best body builder in the world. I was totally devoted to this goal at the expense of my studies. College and Cortland, New York, were not the places to chase my dream.

In December of my freshman year, I called my mother right before finals.

"How's your studying going, Jake?" she asked me.

"Listen Ma, I'm thinking of going to California to pursue body building."

She said, "Hold on a second..."

And she called for my dad.

"Pick up the phone and talk to your kid," I heard her say to my dad, "I'm putting my head in the oven."

I figured I might as well tell them over the phone before I got home so I wouldn't get completely killed.

Well, I reluctantly completed the year. And then, with their blessing, I went to California.

COASTING ON THE COAST

I went out cold to the West Coast. I didn't know a soul. My dad had a business trip to Los Angeles, so I tagged along. He headed back East. I stayed in the West.

I wish I could say it was a glamorous time. But let's face it. I was at the bottom of the food chain. I supported myself by bouncing at a bar.

BUT....

I was in the Mecca of body building. That was a plus. A major plus. At least I was chasing my dream.

And I felt that my family was a big net under me. I could try anything and if I failed, I knew I could go home.

Once again I had thrown myself headfirst into the deep end.

I worked out at the biggest gym in Santa Monica, where all the biggest body builders were working out. No longer was I the largest guy in the gym, the way I was back East. Here I was among the smallest. But I liked that. Challenges only made it better.

One day when I was in the gym, a man from Universal Studios approached me. He told me my facial structure resembled the former Mr. America who starred in the TV program "The Incredible Hulk." He said there was a show at the Universal Studios tour called "The Makeup Show." He wondered if I wanted to be the Incredible Hulk in the theme park show.

I thought, "Come on. Yeah, right."

But they hired me. Call it blind luck. I was in the right place at the right time. I was prepared for that moment. I kept myself in good shape so I would be ready. Ready for what, I wasn't sure.

That job was important in so many ways. It allowed me to "retire" from bouncing in bars. And it was my entry into show business. I didn't have many lines. I growled a lot. But I was having the time of my life.

When the show went off the air, I was out of a job. Now I wondered exactly who I was. Could it be—possibly—that show business or acting was what I wanted? At that point my goal in life had changed in a profound way. Working at Universal Studios opened my eyes and opened many doors for me. I saw a whole other world: the world of show business. It was bursting with exciting possibilities. I knew then that I wanted to be part of that world. In fact, I hungered for it.

CREATING THE PERSONAL TRAINER INDUSTRY

Sometimes opportunity knocks. Other times, it's just a tap. Soon after I lost my job as the Incredible Hulk, opportunity tapped. But I was absolutely ready to move ahead in my life.

An actress I knew was starring in a Club Med commercial. She had to wear a bikini and she wanted to be in superb shape. She wanted me to help her.

"How much are you going to charge me?" she wondered.

I wasn't even thinking about getting paid. "Give me enough for gas money," I replied.

I went to her house and I came up with a 30-minute exercise program. She wasn't entering the Olympics. All she was doing was trying to look good for a TV commercial.

"I need to get in shape," she told me, "but I don't want to look 'pumped up'... like you."

She didn't like weights, which was fine. There are dozens of ways to get into shape. So I improvised with broomsticks and chairs. Instead of pumping iron, I had her pull down on a towel I was holding. That was a great isometric exercise. I kept all the sessions fun and upbeat.

She needed more than my exercise expertise. She also needed to be reassured about her progress. She needed to be motivated to meet her goals. She needed to be kept interested in the program I devised. I found that I was able to meet all those needs easily. I not only shaped her body, I shaped her mind. She left with a positive attitude about herself and the job she was undertaking.

Fortunately, this actress was very well connected in Hollywood. Everyone complimented her on her new, improved figure. "What are you doing to look so good?" they'd ask her. And she told them about me. Then they'd ask for my phone number. Almost overnight, I developed a following.

I'd be out during the day, and when I'd come in and check my answering machine, there'd be messages from people like Steven Spielberg, Priscilla Presley, Harrison Ford, and John Landis. My first big-time client was Margot Kidder when she was doing the *Superman* movies. Once I started training her, It dawned on me that maybe this was a business for me. I liked what I was doing. I was good at it. And I was making some money.

I decided I needed to publicize my work. I approached a public relations expert and told her what I did. I said that I was a "personal trainer" who creates personal exercise programs for people in their homes.

This immediately stoked her interest because it was something totally new.

"Why do you have to train them at home?" she asked. "Why can't you just meet them in a gym?"

"I believe you're the strongest you can be in your own environment," I answered. "You can't be intimidated in your own home. A gym can feel like a metal jungle."

She asked me what my company was called.

I really hadn't thought of a name for my business. Suddenly, I just blurted out, "Body by Jake."

"Very catchy," she replied.

GETTING MY FITNESS BUSINESS IN SHAPE

Life was wonderful to me. Out of nothing, I created a business called personal training. Ten thousand dollars sat in my bank account. Not a fortune, but I wasn't complaining.

I was all set to buy a condominium. But then it struck me. The heck with the condo. I was going to buy a Mercedes-Benz.

I took out $9,400. I put it down on a black Mercedes 380SL. Nervous? You bet. The payments for my car were higher than my apartment. But I said to myself. "They'll take this apartment away before they take this car away."

Hollywood is all about image, and I correctly perceived that this car was going to help put my career in the fast lane. Now, when I pulled up to these people's homes I wasn't the gym instructor anymore. I was a successful *personal trainer and businessman.* I promoted myself.

I also pushed, challenged, and tested myself. With only $600 in the bank, I promised myself that I was going to win. I had to win. I didn't want to lose what I had. And it made me go to the next step.

Once I got that car, every story written about me invariably had this line, "Jake pulls up to his celebrity client's home in his black Mercedes-Benz..."

Sure, it was a material thing. But it made people reevaluate me and perceive that I was successful.

An exercise book was my next step. Why not? I had a winning program. I had a growing public persona. And I had the sizzle of my Hollywood clients. I put together my concept, went to book publishers, and sold my idea. Then I did an exercise video.

These were all entirely new fields for me. I didn't know any of the rules. There wasn't time to be scared. I was constantly challenging myself. And I knew I was going to do well. I just knew it. My ideas were good. My training methods were sound. I had something unique to offer.

It was inevitable that others would come into my field and become personal fitness trainers, too. That was just fine for me. The profession grew under my feet. And that only kept pushing me higher and higher.

MUSCLING INTO THE TV LINEUP

Over the years, I've had lots of cameo roles and small parts in movies like *Coming to America* and *Tough Guys*. But I always wanted to have my own show. This was perhaps the biggest challenge of my career.

After my first exercise video came out in 1984, I was interviewed for a CNN news program. Shortly thereafter, a top CNN executive called and asked me to think of doing some type of exercise show for CNN.

"Like what?" I asked."

"Think of something," he said.

I knew I didn't want to be Jake "LaLanne." I didn't want to be just an exercise guy. I knew in my heart that I was capable of more.

I wanted to conceive something for CNN that would show off my personality, motivate people, and make them smile.

So I came up with "Fitness Break by Jake." These one-minute segments were set at a beautiful location featuring me with two great-looking women. In 60 seconds, I demonstrated one quick fitness tip. It was fun. It was upbeat. It was informative. And to top it off, people all over the world watched it. From 1984 to 1988, these fitness tips ran three times a day.

After "Fitness Break by Jake," I had an idea to do my own half-hour health and fitness show. I teamed up with an entertainment company that was just starting a TV division, and we launched the "Body by Jake" show nationally in 1988. We did 100 episodes and it lasted two years. From there I took my show to ESPN, where "Body by Jake" has been on the air since 1990.

FROM SIT-UPS TO BELLY LAUGHS

In the late 1980s, I created an idea for my own sitcom. I would play the central character—a big brother. I never saw a sitcom where the big brother was in charge of the household. Plus in real life, I was a big brother to my siblings. That's what made it so appealing to me.

I've always felt comfortable setting goals I knew I could accomplish, and I was certain I could play me.

I met with executives at the broadcast networks. They wanted to change my concept and make me a personal trainer and bodyguard to a different celebrity every week. But that wasn't what I envisioned. I wanted to break out of the personal trainer mold. So I said thank you and hunted for another deal.

I was a little discouraged, but I really felt it was their loss. They were missing the boat. That's how much I believed in my idea. All I wanted was an opportunity. If I was no good, they could throw me out.

Nobody got what I was saying until I met with Tim Robertson, president of the Family Channel. He understood immediately and in September 1990, the Family Channel began broadcasting my sitcom, "Big Brother Jake." As of this writing, it's the highest rated original show on the Family Channel.

FROM ME TO YOU

Looking back on these successes, it seems so simple. But I'll never forget that I was told no a million times. It was no-no-no-no-no-no-no-no-no-no-no-no-no-no-no-no-no-no-no-no-no-no-no-no-no-no-no-no-no-no-no-no-no-no-no-no-no-no-no-no-no-no-no.

"No, Jake, you can't do fitness videos with towels and chairs. Everyone's doing aerobics."

"No, Jake, you can't star in a sitcom as a big brother. You have to be a musclehead."

"No, Jake, you can't borrow money from a bank to create your own licensing company. You're a start-up company."

I learned that *no* is not a bad word. It makes you stronger. It makes you work harder. It forces you not to be complacent.

Overcoming the no's made me believe in myself. I don't play the stock market. I only bet on things that I'm sure of.

And now I'm offering you suggestions based on my success as just a regular guy. If you believe in yourself, you can do it. Hey look, it

14 takes a lot of work and a lot of sweat. But if you really want it and you believe in yourself, you can do it.

Just remember:

DON'T QUIT!

So how do you get started? What does it take to change your attitude, your routine, and ultimately your life? As you'll discover in the following chapters, you start one day at a time.

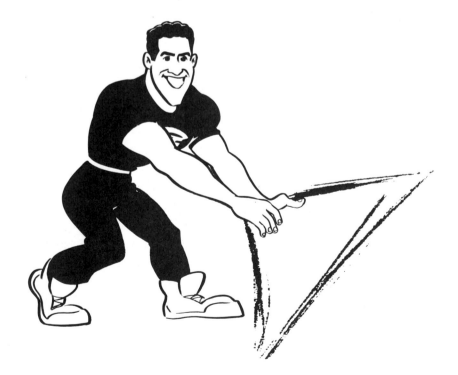

THE MORNING PUMP

The Morning Pump is about:

■ Motivation
■ Organization
■ Exercise
■ Preparing your body and your mind for the day.

The morning pump is a time of beginnings and fresh opportunities. It's a time to reshape your body and your mind. Forget about yesterday. Today is a new day, and this morning is your first chance at making it a great day.

So that's why the MORNING PUMP is always at the top of my list. It's my time to *get motivated*, *get organized*, *get energized*, and *get ready* for the day ahead.

Sounds good, right?

That's how I start my day. Every day. And here's how I do it.

GET UP EARLY!

I do two things to make sure I'm never behind in the morning. First I get up *real* early: 5:20 A.M. Second, I set my watch 20 minutes fast. So even though my alarm goes off at 5:20, it's really 5:00 A.M. The result?

I'm never late for *anything*.

My father used to tell me that there's always someone going to bed a little later and getting up a little earlier than me just to keep me motivated. So I used to go to bed at 11 P.M. and rise at 2:30 A.M. Unless someone was an insomniac, there was no way *anyone* was going to sleep fewer hours than me. What's the old saying about the early bird getting the worm? Well, I want the *whole* worm...every day.

I still get to bed at 11 P.M. But now I rise at 5 A.M. It may *sound* early, but I need this jump on the day to be sure everything runs in stride. This way I'm able to exercise, eat a healthy breakfast, read the newspaper, make a phone call to my Body by Jake Licensing Corporation, talk to my assistant in L.A., and read through the current "Big Brother Jake" script—*all* before I head off to the studio for a full day's work. By the time I'm in the car,

- I'm *relaxed*.
- I'm *pumped* for the day.
- And I'm *ahead of schedule*.

Now, a lot went on from the time I opened my eyes to the time I popped into the car. It's my morning ritual—my MORNING PUMP. Again, it's about motivation, organization, and exercise. It's what keeps me pumped all day and ensures me a sense of efficiency and control. It works great for me in my own way, and it can work just as good for you in your own way.

When the alarm goes off, sit up in bed and immediately think, "It's going to be a great day." (A word on alarms here. Alarming is just what they shouldn't be. Turn off that annoying buzzer. Try a soothing music radio station, instead.) Reinforce this concept of a great day. Actually say it to yourself with conviction: "It's going to be a great day. It's going to be a great day."

This will create a positive frame of mind first thing in the morning, which will last throughout the day.

Remember:

POSITIVE THINGS HAPPEN TO POSITIVE PEOPLE.

As your eyes become focused, look at your list.

List? That's right. Your things-to-do list. The one you wrote last night listing everything you need to accomplish today. This is one of the true fundamentals of mental fitness. It lightens the load in your mind. Instead of carrying around a million things to do, you've written them down—it's out of your head and onto the page. You won't have to waste any energy remembering what it was that you told yourself to do twelve hours ago. You can direct your energies toward more productive and enjoyable things.

I'm a real fan of creating lists. It's something I do every night (for more on making lists, see Chapter 5). I put it on the table next to my bed so it's the first thing I see when I wake up. This list becomes my *game plan* for the day. It's my compass that points me in the right direction for the next eighteen hours. This list is golden!

As the day progresses and things get accomplished, those accomplishments get *checked off* the list and *checked out* of your mind.

Should something unexpected happen that isn't on your list, you're able to direct your energies toward it and then redirect them back to your list. This way, you're still on course.

One final note about notes: The items that aren't checked off I just write on tomorrow's list. And then I take that checked-off list and move it to another drawer where I keep all my things-to-do for the month. At the end of the month, I pull out all thirty or so lists and examine what I've accomplished. Talk about feeling great about yourself!

EXERCISE

You bet!

Exercise is one of the major parts of my ritual that sets my day straight. When I'm working out, with each repetition I do I try to relate to something I have to accomplish during the day. So by the time I've finished all my reps and all the sets, I have *physically* worked my body, and have *mentally* completed everything on my list. Now my mind and body are prepared for the day.

It works for me. And I know it can work for you. Plus, think of all the great perks you get from exercising:

- You're able to slide your skirt on easier.
- Your short-sleeve shirt looks pretty sporty after working the ol' bi-mans (biceps).
- You stand up straight and walk with confidence.
- You're axin' the *weight* and feelin' *great*!

WHEN YOU FEEL GOOD ABOUT YOURSELF, OTHERS WILL FEEL GOOD ABOUT YOU, TOO.

I'm talking from experience here. And the morning is the best time of the day to exercise because...

1. You're more rested in the morning.
2. You'll be energized for an entire day.
3. It's out of the way for the rest of the day.

What it boils down to is that exercise gets your heart pumping, gets your metabolism going, helps you burn more calories, and gets your mind *psyched*!

To get you in gear, I've created a special exercise program that you'll find in Chapter 7. But before you do anything, keep reading.

TAKE A MEETING...WITH YOURSELF

Find the best mirror in your home. Personally, I prefer the bathroom mirror because I can shut the door and look at myself squarely in the mirror. Direct eye contact. Jake on Jake. I talk to myself about what I'm doing that day and what I want to accomplish.

This gets me psyched. I'm thinking all the time as I'm shaving, "It's a brand new day. Whatever happened yesterday—good, bad, or indifferent—I've still got a fresh start *today*. And I'm going to make the best of it whether it's a big deal or a small meeting."

BE BRIEF ▪ BE TOUGH ▪ BE HONEST

It's a pat on my back and a kick in my buttisimo. And it gets me in gear. This is also a good time to recite the "Don't Quit" poem which you'll read on the next page. Tape it on the bathroom mirror so you can see it while you're shaving or applying your makeup.

"DON'T QUIT"

When things go wrong as they sometimes will,
When the road you're trudging seems all uphill,
When the funds are low, and the debts are high,
And you want to smile, but you have to sigh,
When care is pressing you down a bit,
Rest, if you must, but do not quit.

Life is queer, with its twists and turns
As every one of us sometimes learns.
And many a failure turns about
When he might have won had he stuck it out.
Don't give up, though the pace seems slow.
You may succeed with another blow.

Success is failure turned inside out—
The silver tint of the clouds of doubt.
And you never can tell how close you are.
It may be near when it seems so far.
So stick to the fight when you're hardest hit.
It's when things seem worst that you must not quit.

JAKE'S FAVORITE FIVE PLACES TO PUT HIS "DON'T QUIT" POEM
    Night table
    Fridge
    Wallet or pocketbook
    Bathroom mirror
    Under the computer keypad
JAKE'S BONUS LOCATION
    In the cookie jar

COMMUNICATION

Talk to your spouse, a good friend, or pet about what you're going to accomplish that day. My wife and I like to talk every morning about the day ahead of us. Being able to bounce ideas off your teammate gives you more confidence.

YOU ARE A WINNER...SO EAT LIKE ONE!

Light makes right.

After I exercise, I eat bran cereal with skim milk and fruit, a bagel, a large orange juice, and some water. Get the picture?

I stay away from donuts, pastries, bacon, and other fattening foods. They may get you pumped up for a while, but they're going to slow you down in the long run. If you need a little pump-up in the morning, walk a few flights of stairs on your way into the office, take the dog on a longer walk, or park you car further from the market.

Fuel up every morning. Your body is like a finely tuned automobile engine. It needs proper upkeep and good fuel like fruits, grains, and vegetables to run smoothly.

STAY TUNED IN

HOW CAN YOU EXPECT TO CONQUER THE DAY IF YOU DON'T EVEN KNOW WHAT'S GOING ON OUTSIDE YOUR FRONT DOOR?

Whether you skim the newspaper while you're eating breakfast or watch a morning news program as you're getting dressed in the morning, *keep informed* of the events taking place in your world. An article you read in the morning might help you in the office or home. It's a winning way to start the day.

I try to get as much information as possible before I start making my business calls. Television's morning news programs give me a complete world roundup in five minutes. I also breeze through at least two newspapers in the morning. My motto: be *tuned in* to the outside world before you *step out* the front door.

IN A NUTSHELL:

- You've gone over your list.
- You've recited the "Don't Quit" poem.
- You've fueled up on a healthy breakfast.
- You're informed.
- You're feeling positive about yourself and your upcoming day.

Now you're in charge of the day, and the day's not in charge of you!

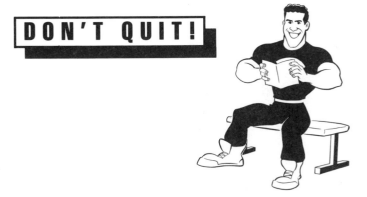

DON'T QUIT!

THE MIDDAY KICKER

Midday is the swing time in your day. It's a transitional period when you can turn a good day into a great day. For that, you should be alert, confident, and productive.

It's the time to kick into high gear. You know what I mean. Just a little tap on the ol' buttisimo to keep your engines revved. That's why I call this section the MIDDAY KICKER. In the midday, you need to:

- Stay focused.
- Stay pumped.
- Stay on target.

Your goal is to maximize this crucial part of the day. And here's how you do it.

STICK TO YOUR LIST

Priority 1. I can't emphasize this enough. Your list is your compass for the day. Refer to it constantly, especially at midday. This way you can get a sense of what you've accomplished and what needs to be done.

IF YOU CAN SEE IT, YOU CAN FOCUS ON IT!

Having that list in front of you gives you an added sense of direction and eliminates distraction. I go over my list a hundred times during the day.

Challenge yourself to complete the list.

OLD BUSINESS
1. Don't forget stamps
2. Call Fred
3. Re-schedule appointment with dentist

NEW BUSINESS
1. 6 a.m. workout
2. Make restaurant reservation
3. Do draft of budget report
4. MILK!
5. Get dry cleaning
6. Call accountant

CLEAR THE DECK

Before you leave for lunch, straighten your work area (desk, kitchen, car, etc.). Just taking five minutes to clean up is one of the most productive things you can do in the middle of the day. Here's why:

1. A clutter-free desk makes for a clutter-free mind.
2. It gives you a sense of control because everything is in its place.
3. You will jump right back into your day when you return from lunch without having to sift through a mound of papers.

I always clean my desk before I leave for lunch. I'm not only *physically* putting things away, I'm clearing it mentally as well.

Even if you don't work in an office, it's still important to maintain order. For example, if you work in your kitchen, make sure all the dishes are put away and the counters are clean. Or if you work out of your car, throw away the morning paper and crumpled coffee cup.

The minutes it takes to get your work area in shape will probably save you hours later in the week. My time—and your time—is precious!

MAKE LUNCHTIME THE RIGHT TIME

Lunch is the "half time" in your working day. If you've worked hard all morning, you're probably already running on near-empty and looking forward to grabbing a bite to eat. But remember:

MAKE LUNCHTIME MORE FULFILLING.

Lunch is a time to *recharge* your body and *refocus* your mind. Don't miss a lunch even if you lead an active, busy life. Carve out at least 30 minutes for lunch. Use this time to:

- Relax.
- Reflect on the morning.
- Redirect your energy for the rest of the day.

A word about lunchtime food. As long as you're smart and sensible, you can eat nutritiously practically anywhere. Look for foods high in protein and low in fat. Fish and poultry are excellent lunchtime choices. I prefer skinless chicken, tuna (in water) on whole wheat bread, salads, and pastas.

Like breakfast, your goal is to stay light. Aim to leave the lunch table energized, not bogged down.

GET PHYSICAL!

After lunch, you may be mentally prepared but your body can still feel sluggish. So before you get back into the swing of your day, do some light exercise.

You won't break a sweat here. You'll just restart your engines, get the wheels turning again, and loosen those muscles.

Close the door to your office and/or the blinds to your home and do the exercises on the following pages.

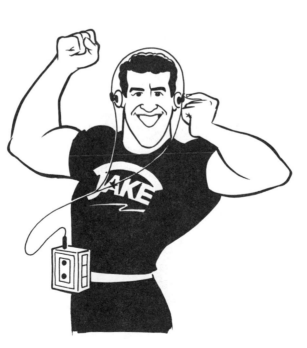

NECK ROLL

Begin in the Jake stance. (Feet shoulder-width apart. Knees slightly bent. Buttisimo and stomach are tight.) Keep your hands fisted and slightly flexed.

Slowly drop your head in front of you. Then bring your head to the right side and stretch.

Bring your head back to the center, and then over to the left side for a stretch. (Do these for 1 minute.)

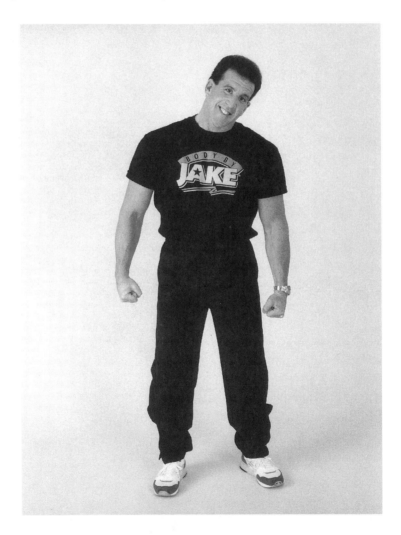

WHEEL ROLL

Begin in the Jake stance. Keeping your arms and hands flexed, roll your arms making big circular motions. Go front ten and back ten.

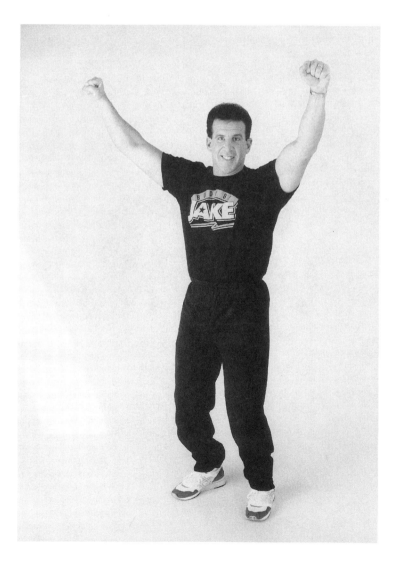

LEG KICK-OUT IN CHAIR

Begin with your back straight and arms flexed tight. Bring legs in toward chest and kick out. Breathe out while you're kicking your legs out.
   Great for lower stomach! (10 reps)

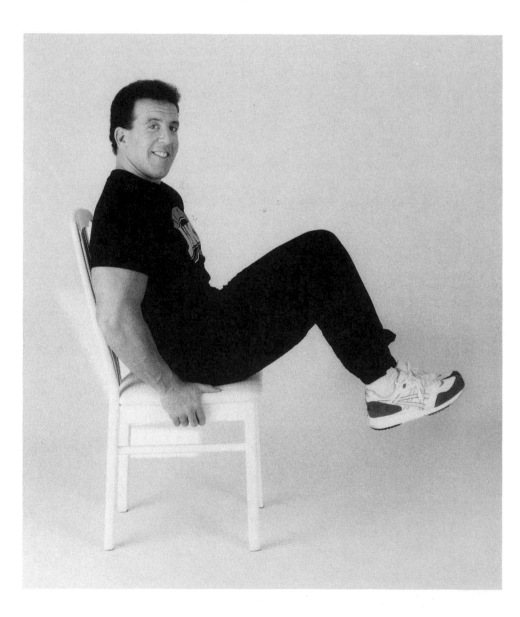

PUSH-UP OFF CHAIR OR DESK

This exercise uses a chair or desk for support. With your back flat and your legs extended, lower the body push-up style to the chair or desk. Be sure not to go all the way down or lock-out your elbows. Breathe normally. (10 reps)

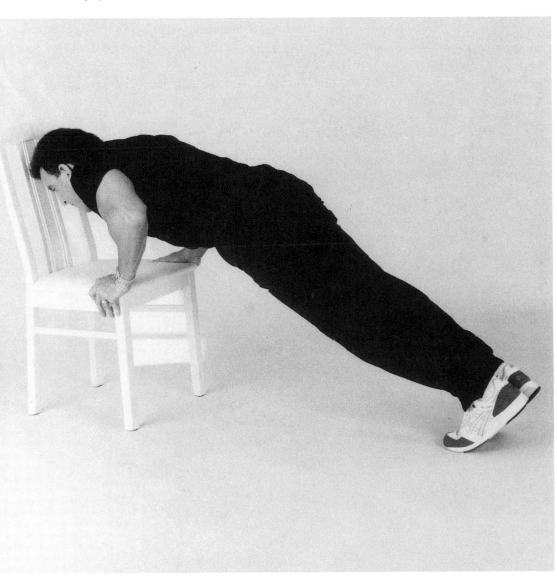

SCISSOR OFF CHAIR

Sitting on the edge of the chair, grip your hands on the edges of the chair.
Leaning slightly back to flex the stomach muscles, extend your legs out in front of you, feet flexed, cross left over right and then right over left.
Be sure to keep the body tight. (10 reps)

I also recommend taking a few office laps or trips up and down your staircase. Again, this helps to work the kinks out of your muscles and refocuses your mind.

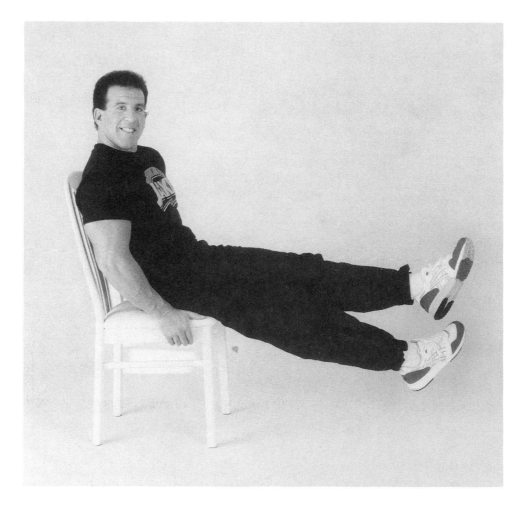

Everyone needs to chalk up some wins in the day. Whether they're small successes or of great magnitude, view every accomplishment as a win. Success breeds more success. It builds confidence. It creates a positive attitude.

So build a series of easy-to-attain goals into your day. For instance:

1. Get the kids to school on time.
2. Rewrite your résumé.
3. Go food shopping for the week.
4. Get to work 10 minutes early and clean out some files.

Will attaining these small goals fulfill your lifetime ambitions? Not directly. But they're important in developing positive feelings about your daily life. And those feelings of accomplishment and success are the building blocks you need to ultimately achieve the major goals in your life.

COMMUNICATE

Have productive conversations with your co-workers, spouse, or friends during the day. This allows you to redirect yourself, focus your attention, and attain your goals. And communication with trusted business associates or friends is essential during the inevitable challenges that arise.

A SHARED CHALLENGE IS HALF A CHALLENGE!

Every day I talk to almost everyone within my circle of friends and business associates. Therefore, everyone knows what's going on and what we're trying to accomplish. Everyone has the same up-to-date information.

Being connected to others who share the same positive attitude I have gives me tremendous emotional power. I listen carefully to what they're saying. They may have a different perspective on a business challenge. They may have that nugget of information I'm looking for. Or they get me thinking about my next big project. They help validate my ideas. They open up blind spots. They make the wins sweeter and the losses easier to tolerate.

From personal experience, I know that creativity and productivity don't develop in a vacuum. They're nurtured through interaction and communication with many people working together as a team.

IN A NUTSHELL, the MIDDAY KICKER is your time to:

■ Stick to your list.
■ Remain organized.
■ Boost your productivity.
■ Refuel your body and refocus your mind.

Your goal is what I call Twin Peaks: Get a *peak* performance at the *peak* of the day!

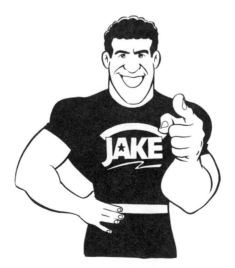

THE EVENING
PEP TALK

The afternoon is drawing to a close. Your work day is almost over. It's now time for the EVENING PEP TALK.

This is when I *review* my day's accomplishments and *preview* tomorrow's game plan. I'm my own coach during the EVENING PEP TALK. I talk to myself as coach to player. It's my time to regroup, rethink, and recharge myself.

You will do the same. Try thinking of the end of the day as a time to look at yourself and your accomplishments honestly. When you're disengaged from the rush of daily activities, it becomes possible to really assess what you've done in the hours since your alarm clock went off. Identify your achievements. Examine any challenges that you may not have overcome. Analyze the choices and decisions you made in the day. During the EVENING PEP TALK, it's also important to take yourself through a physical and mental cool-down routine.

The EVENING PEP TALK is a time for:

■ Introspection
■ Inspiration
■ Relaxation
■ Preparation

35

Like the MORNING PUMP and MIDDAY KICKER, the emphasis of the EVENING PEP TALK is positive. I want you to keep on building on today's accomplishments to reach tomorrow's goals. Here's the plan that I follow.

DO LOOK BACK

The EVENING PEP TALK is the time to ease on the brakes and reflect on what happened during the day. This is the slow-down part of the EVENING PEP TALK.

I always review my day's work at the end of business hours. This gives me a sense of perspective on the day. It allows me to analyze my achievements a step removed from the hectic pace of working hours.

RUSH, RUSH, RUSH, RUSH, RUSH

We all lead busy lives. And for working moms and dads, the end of the day sometimes seems even *more* hectic than regular business hours. But it's still possible (and very desirable) to find a few quiet moments for reflection. These "moments" are all around you. You just have to find them.

For instance, think about your day as you're coming home from work, when you're returning from a late-afternoon errand, or even when you're washing up for dinner. You don't need a lot of time. The main thing is to block off just a few private minutes so you can have your own personal pep talk.

CONFRONT YOURSELF!

Ask yourself these two key questions:

1. What did I accomplish today?
2. How can I build on what I learned today?

I'm not just talking about making big changes in your personal life or closing huge deals. Perhaps you cooked a new meal for your family. Ask them what they liked about it, and use their comments to create a new dish for next week's dinner. Maybe you made a great suggestion at a staff meeting in the office. Now's the time to think about the follow-through. These are worthy achievements. It's important to develop a daily routine of identifying them and building on them. Don't forget to look over your list to help you recall the day's accomplishments.

Be candid with yourself. Be analytical. But overall, be positive.

GIVE YOURSELF A BREAK

In other words...relax.

Relaxation is a key ingredient in a successful daily routine. Everybody—myself included—needs to ease up at the end of the day. It's important to focus on activities outside your daily work routine.

I devote at least an hour every day to relaxation. I take a walk, ride a bike, or play basketball. Another favorite form of relaxation for me is making a salad. The simple routine of peeling carrots, chopping celery, and washing the lettuce gives me enormous pleasure. I find these easy physical tasks a soothing and productive way to release tension and redirect my energy from the day. And when I'm under lots of stress, you should see the salads I make!

Spending quality time with your family is a good way to relax. Forget about a three-course dinner for tonight. Instead, pick up a take-out dinner and take the kids to a nearby park. Leisure time with your family is a significant part of your day. Also, when you take a few moments to talk over the day with family and friends, it sometimes puts your successes and challenges in the proper perspective. And that clarifies your thinking as you begin to proceed with tomorrow's game plan.

There's another important element to this part of the day: *personal growth*. It's easy to slip into the same relaxation routines every night. Look at the early evening as a time for expanding your mind and developing your body. Sure, it's OK to "veg out" once in a while. But relaxation does not necessarily mean the absence of productive activity. The EVENING PEP TALK should be a high point of the day for personal growth. And that growth is only going to happen if you actively push yourself. So be creative.

Challenge yourself to do something out of character. For instance, I never used to go to museums. When I pushed myself to go (and believe me, it was out of character), I began to enjoy it. That's a growth experience.

Here are some suggestions for you to consider:

Go to the library.
Cook a gourmet meal.
Take a walk.
Volunteer your time for a worthwhile cause.
Watch the sunset.
Take an adult-education course.
Learn to play a musical instrument.
Attend a concert.
Read a book.
Master a new sport like ice skating or paddle-tennis.
Plant some flowers.
Wash your car.
Write someone a letter.

THE B-I-G LIST

Psssst! Wanna know the secret of a successful day?

This is it. Your things-to-do list. Don't end today without making a new one for tomorrow.

It's your compass, your Bible, your pointer, your life raft, your signpost—whatever you want to call it. For me, it's the whole enchilada. Nothing is more important in my daily workday routine. Having the list allows me to operate at peak efficiency. It clarifies my thinking. It sharpens my mental vision.

The preparation of the list marks a *big* turning point in your day. It means you've put today's business behind you and now you're ready to focus on tomorrow's.

WHAT YOU PLAN TONIGHT WILL HAPPEN TOMORROW.

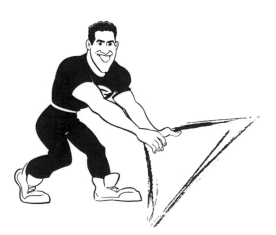

That's why making a list is so important. Take a few minutes to compose your things-to-do list. Clear your head. Get a clean sheet of paper. Concentrate on everything you want to accomplish in your professional and personal life. Consider these main points:

■ *Start the new day with old business.*
The loose ends you didn't tie up today should be the first things to address tomorrow.

■ *Make your list in order of importance.*
In other words, prioritize!
    After old business, the day's most significant calls and activities belong at the top of your list. For the real important business, I suggest red ink so it really pops off the page.

■ *Include starting-block goals.*
Write down two or three tasks that will be easily achieved. This will give you a sense of accomplishment, no matter what happens during the day. These goals might include washing the car, picking up dry cleaning, or filing an expense account.

■ *Include telephone numbers.*
This eliminates wasted time scrambling through your phone book to find someone's number.

■ *Include the purpose of your call.*
It's easy to forget why we're calling someone. When you write down the reason for your call, it will help keep your conversation short and to the point.

■ *Leave room for notes.*
This way, your list (which you'll save) becomes a useful reference tool to recall conversations and meetings.

SAVE YOUR LISTS

This is important. Every few weeks, take a look at your lists. It's a great way to chart your accomplishments and feel positive about yourself!

OLD BUSINESS
1. Don't forget stamps ✓
2. Call Fred (done)
3. Re-schedule appointment with dentist ✓

NEW BUSINESS
1. 6 a.m. workout
2. Make restaurant reservation
3. Do draft of budget report
4. MILK!
5. Get dry cleaning
6. Call accountant

On the pages that follow, you'll see an example of what *your* things-to-do list should look like.

THINGS TO DO

TODAY'S DATE_____

MY GOAL TODAY IS_____

OLD BUSINESS

Completed

1.   ☐

Phone number_____

Date_____

Notes_____

_____

2.   ☐

Phone number_____

Date_____

Notes_____

_____

3.   ☐

Phone number_____

Date_____

Notes_____

_____

NEW BUSINESS

1.
Completed ☐

Phone number_____

Date_____

Notes_____

_____

2.
☐

Phone number_____

Date_____

Notes_____

_____

3.
☐

Phone number_____

Date_____

Notes_____

_____

4.
☐

Phone number_____

Date_____

Notes_____

_____

DON'T QUIT!

HAVE A FINE DINE

You've been eating well all day. There's no reason to break away from your successful and healthy eating routine. Some great dinner ideas include pastas, chicken, salads, fish, fruits, vegetables, and lean cuts of beef and pork. Even treat yourself to a light dessert. Angel food cake with fruit is a healthy choice. I frequently enjoy a cup of cappuccino at night. In fact, you don't have to starve or deny yourself at dinnertime. But remember: moderation is important.

Try to eat between 6 and 8 P.M. If you eat late in the evening, the food will just lay in your stomach overnight. Not only will you feel sluggish in the morning but it's a surefire way to put on some unwanted pounds.

EAT LIGHT TONIGHT TO FEEL RIGHT TOMORROW.

GET UP FOR YOUR COOL DOWN

Pre-bedtime exercise is a great way to relax. In the morning, you exercise to get the engines revved. In the afternoon, you re-energize yourself with a few exercises. Now it's time to s-t-r-e-t-c-h yourself—literally. Stretching relaxes your muscles and keeps you limber. It helps relieve tension.

The purpose of evening exercise is to cool down physically and mentally from your day. I just want you to soothe your mind and loosen your muscles. Do it while listening to music or watching television. A few stretches that I like to do are on the following pages.

Hold each stretch for at least ten seconds.
Relax into the movement.

ARE YOU READY TO S-T-R-E-T-C-H?

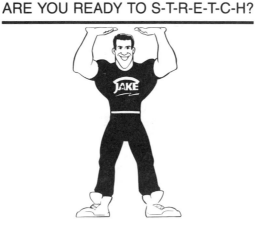

WISHBONE STRETCH

Sitting on the ground with your legs wide apart, knees slightly bent, begin with your body in the center and facing forward.

Slowly reach out in front of you, breathing out as you reach forward. Don't Bounce.

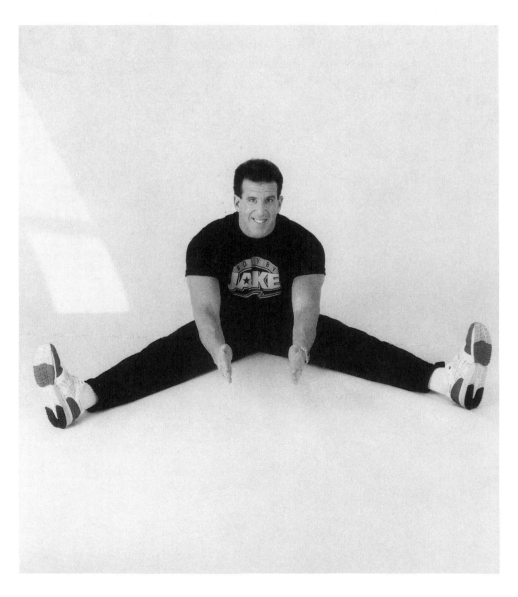

Bring the arms and body over to the left, reaching toward your toes. And *then over to the right.*

This stretches the sides, lower back, upper back, and hamstrings. Great stress reliever!

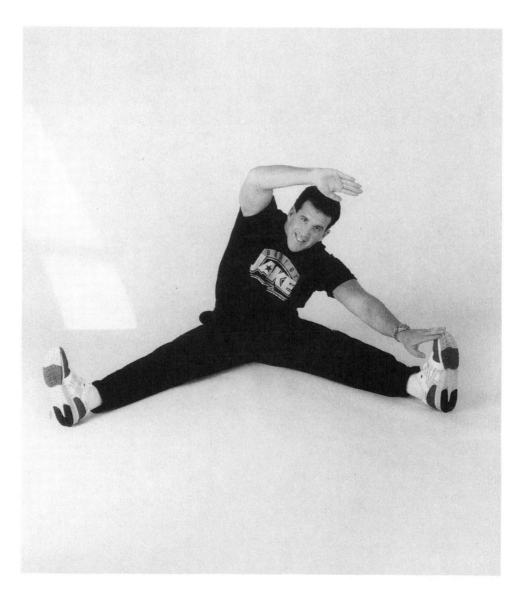

INVERTED HURDLE

Begin with your right leg extended. Bend your left leg so that your left leg lies on the ground and your left foot touches your right leg.

Stretch the body out toward your right toe.

Change legs.

Breathe out and reach out.

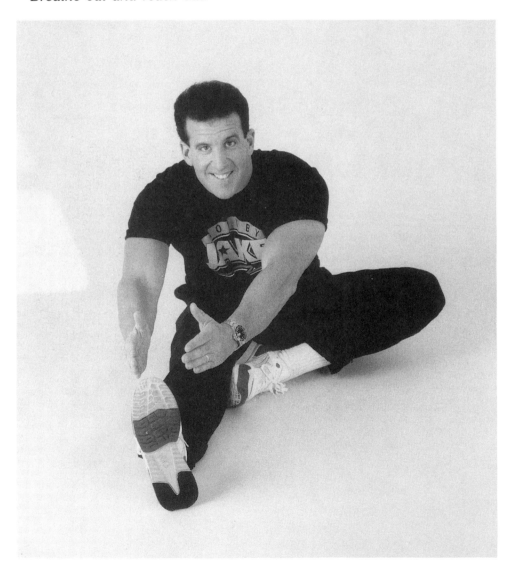

WALLET STRETCH

Knees bent slightly, reach over toward your toes, breathing out as you reach out.

This is a great stretch for hamstrings, and the lower back.

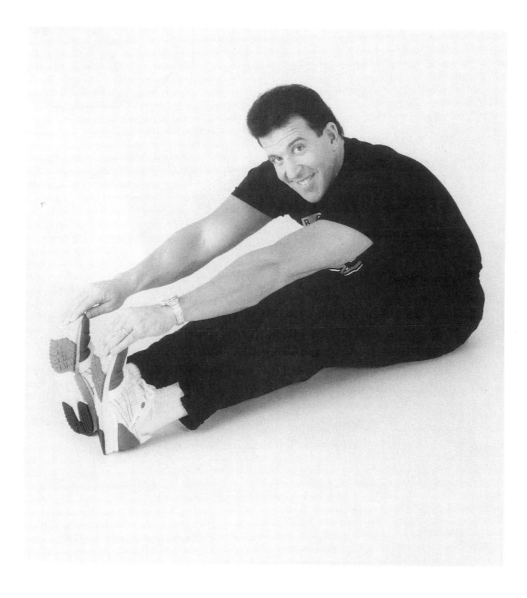

POW-WOW STRETCH

Begin in a pow-wow sit with your knees bent and your feet facing toward each other.

Letting the inner thighs stretch, roll your head forward, stretching your upper and lower back as well as the inner thighs.

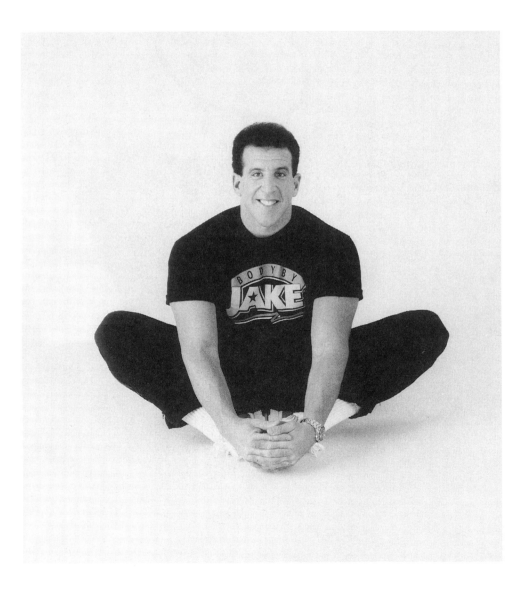

ROLL-UP STRETCH

Begin by standing up straight and tall.
Cross the legs, one over the other.
Bending from the waist, roll forward reaching for your toes. Knees are slightly bent as you roll, and be sure to breathe normally.
Slowly roll back up and change legs.

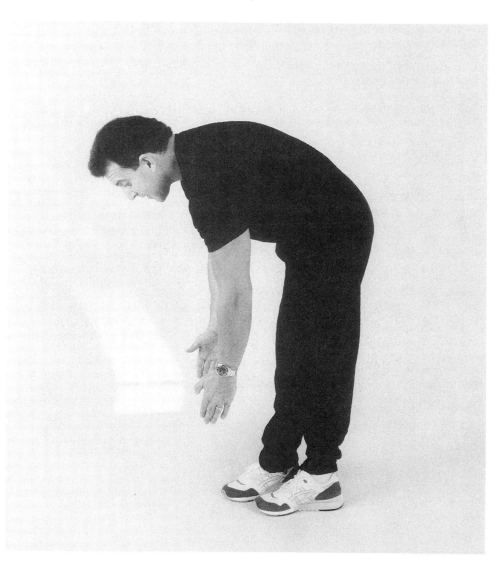

SET YOURSELF UP FOR TOMORROW

Imagine rising early in the morning after a good night's sleep with a sense of purpose and direction. Better yet, picture yourself in the morning routine as crisp, efficient, and containing no surprises. (If you ever woke up in the morning to find there was no coffee or bread in the house, you know what I mean.)

Sounds like a good picture, right?

Organization in the morning begins with preparation in the evening. I get ready for my sunrise routine *before* I go to sleep to make sure my new day starts smoothly. To have an easy morning, follow these nighttime tips:

1. Check the weather forecast. This will help determine your clothes for the day.

2. Pick the clothes you'll wear. (And if you have young kids, choose their clothes as well.)

3. Iron your clothes (if necessary).

4. Make sure there's milk, juice, and bread in the house.

5. Find your car keys. Place them next to your wallet or in your pocketbook.

6. Put your wallet or pocketbook in same spot every night.

7. Pack your bag (or briefcase, gym bag, or school knapsack).

8. Stick your things-to-do list on your night table so it's the first thing you see in the morning.

These are simple and obvious nighttime tips. Follow them each night and you'll be surprised at how this new routine will improve your morning efficiency.

IN A NUTSHELL, the EVENING PEP TALK is a time to:

■ Create your things-to-do list.
■ Identify the positive points of the day.
■ Build on your accomplishments.
■ Stretch your muscles, soothe your mind.
■ Relax.
■ Prepare for the next day.

REVIEW TODAY, RELAX TONIGHT, AND CONQUER TOMORROW.

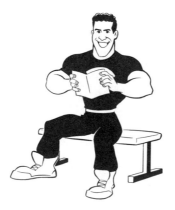

WEEKENDS

You've made it.

The weekend. The time of the week just for *you*. Right?

Maybe.

In theory, the weekend should be a time for relaxation, regrouping, and reenergizing yourself. That's the ideal way to spend the weekend.

In practice, weekends can place a lot of demands on you. It's the time to catch up with your family, take care of the car, get groceries, mow the lawn, balance the checkbook, watch the Little League game, visit friends and relatives, clean the basement, and engage in other assorted errands. And if you're like me, you probably brought home some office projects to work on during your "spare" time over the weekend.

Whew! Weekends can be exhausting. Active, productive people often carry a lot of responsibilities. But we also have a responsibility to *take care of ourselves* on the weekend. Remember:

YOUR OVERALL WEEKEND GOAL IS TO MAXIMIZE YOUR RELAXATION AND MINIMIZE YOUR STRESS.

So how do you attain these goals without neglecting your personal and professional duties? I have several suggestions.

TAKE TWO

Block out two hours for just yourself on the weekend. Take a bike ride. See a movie. Go clothes shopping. Leave the kids with a baby-sitter. It's your time. Happy, creative people often need this time off to function more effectively in their daily routines. This also helps prevent burnout—as a parent, a partner, and a breadwinner.

If you can take more time off, fine. But two hours should be the minimum to shoot for.

CATCH UP ON YOUR SLEEP

Sleep the extra hour Saturday and Sunday mornings. If that's difficult, try napping later in the day. If you have small children who rise early, take a nap when they sleep in the afternoon. Or alternate lazy mornings with your spouse: he sleeps late Saturday; she gets off Sunday. Those few minutes of rest during the weekend will pay off in extra hours of energy during the week.

MAINTAIN TIES WITH FRIENDS AND FAMILY

Visit friends or relatives on the weekend. In our rushed daily lives, these relationships may suffer. The weekend is the time to renew these bonds. These relationships give our lives a deeper, fuller meaning.

THROW A CURVE IN YOUR EXERCISE ROUTINE

The weekend is the time to break out of your normal exercise routine. If you want to concentrate more on your regular exercises, that's fine. But Saturday and Sunday are perfect for more "social" exercising. Get involved in volleyball, softball, or basketball games. Instead of going to the movies, take the family rollerblading or biking. Take up sailing. Each of these activities is so pleasurable that it hardly feels like exercise. But they're all great for your body and a terrific way to relax.

PREPARE FOR THE WEEK

Sunday night should be the time to view the week in the most positive light possible. There's no reason to dread Monday or any other day. But let's face it: we've all felt slightly overwhelmed at times Sunday night when facing the chores of the week. But you can avoid those worries by following these two steps:

1. Work on tomorrow's responsibilities today. In other words, during the weekend try to address all the nagging little chores that burden you during the week. For instance, cook and freeze two dinners for the week. Iron a week's worth of outfits. Make sure there's plenty of food in the house. What you accomplish on your weekend will make your week easier. And that will make you more relaxed on Sunday night.

2. Write down your major goals and responsibilities for the week. The ideal time to do this is Sunday night, when you've begun following your routines for the EVENING PEP TALK. Your weekend is winding down. And you've started winding up for the upcoming week. But as you make up your things-to-do list, include an overall goal for the week. It may be something like, "Begin search for a new house" or "Investigate opportunities for part-time business." The objective is to give you a big target to aim for as you steam through the week. The details of how you hit that target are specifically outlined in your daily things-to-do list. But writing down your goals or challenges in clear, concise language helps relieve the burden of carrying it in your head on Sunday night. You're literally pushing it out of your mind onto a piece of paper. And that will make you feel in control.

Sunday nights should be as positive and upbeat as every other night of the week. You're rested and relaxed. You're looking forward to Monday and the rest of the week. You know what you're doing and where you're heading. You have one important thought in your mind.

IT'S GOING TO BE A GREAT WEEK. DON'T QUIT!

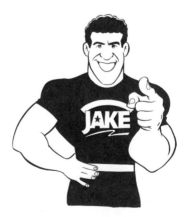

JAKE'S BIG TEN: PHYSICAL EXERCISES

Fitness begins in the mind. And to get your mind in shape, the best place to start is with some body work. Together, a strong mind and a strong body create the chemistry for success. After all, it's easier to feel good about yourself when you're physically fit.

That's why in the next two chapters I introduce you to my "big ten" in both areas: ten top physical exercises to keep your body trim and toned up; ten top mind exercises that help you mentally muscle your way to the top.

Before attempting any of the following physical exercises—or, for that matter, any new exercise program—be sure to check with a doctor.

For exercises with free weights, women should use 3- to 5-pound weights; men should use 10- to 15-pound weights. Aim for 20 repetitions each and build from there. Take it at your own pace. Have fun. And always challenge yourself!

1. THE BIG REACH

Start in the Jake stance. (Feet shoulder-width apart. Knees slightly bent. Buttisimo and stomach are tight.) With the palms facing toward each other, reach up to the sky, one arm at a time, left then right. (That's 1 rep) Alternate arms. This exercise really gets the blood flowing. Breathe normally.

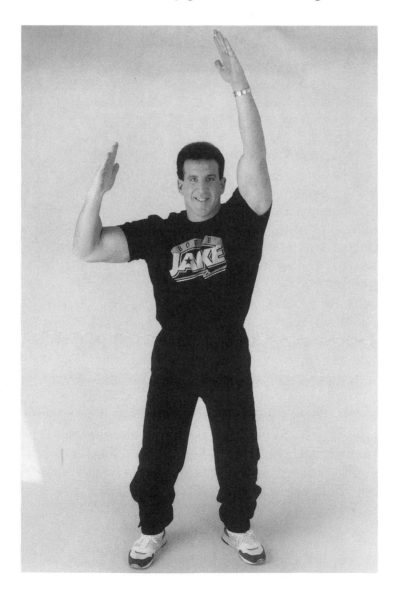

2. SMALL TWIST

Start in the Jake stance. Head is facing forward. Hands fisted and chest high, gently twist to each side. Don't twist all the way around. Keep the motion small and tight. This is an easy twist, just to get our muscles loosened up. This is a great exercise for the waist, hips, and lower back.

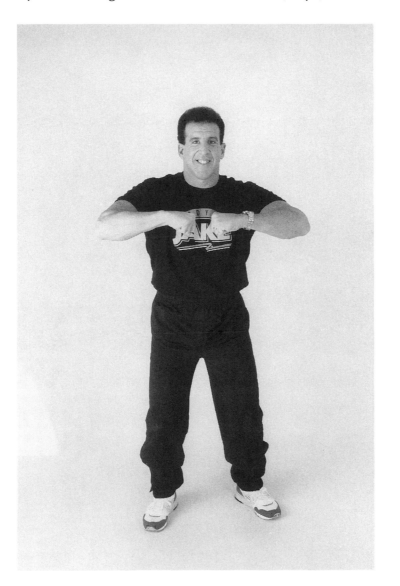

3. JAKE RUN

Begin with your palms on the ground, hands shoulder-width apart, elbows slightly bent and your back flat. Bend your right leg in toward the chest and extend left leg. Exchange the legs, making sure not to bounce or arch your back. Stay as low to the ground as you can. This gives your entire body a wonderful workout. This exercise benefits the whole body.

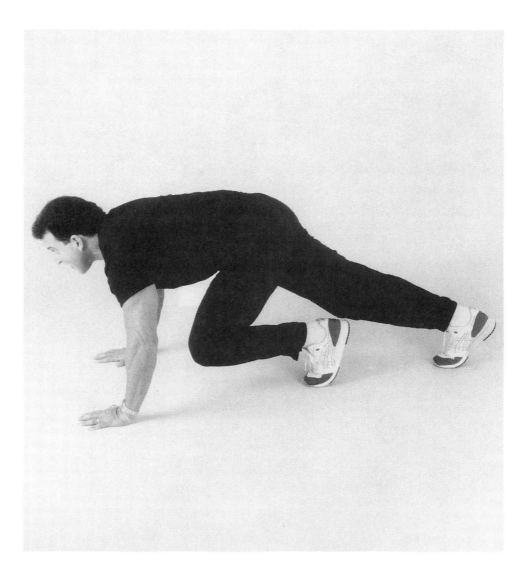

4. POP PUSH-UP

Knees are bent on the ground. Hands are shoulder-width apart. Palms are on the ground. Back is flat. Using the knees as a fulcrum, roll forward as you go down, being sure not to lock out the elbows. This is a great exercise for chest, arms, and shoulders.

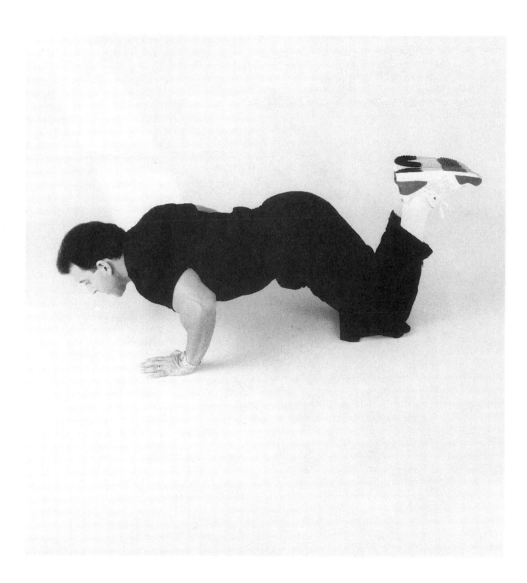

5. SHOULDER PRESS

Start in the Jake stance. With a pair of weights (two cans of Momma's tomato paste are also just fine) bring your arms to shoulder height. With palms facing forward, lift up. Don't lock out the elbows. Bring the weights back to shoulder height. Excellent for shoulders.

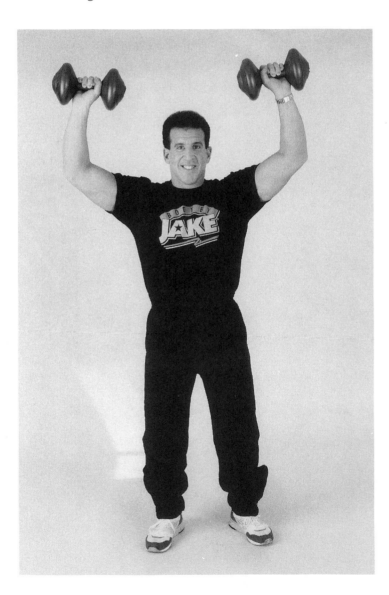

6A. BEGINNER SIT-UP

Start with your back flat on the ground, knees bent and shoulder-width apart. Palms face each other as you reach through your knees. Breathe out as you reach through. Be sure to keep those shoulders off the ground and chin off the chest. Get ready for a flat stomach!

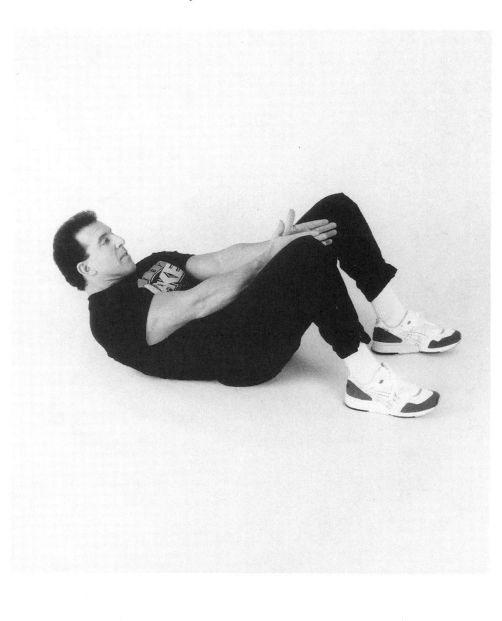

6B. SCRUNCH

Start with your back flat on the ground. Bend your knees in toward your chest. With your shoulders off the ground and your hands against your ears, reach your elbows to your knees while breathing out, as you reach up.

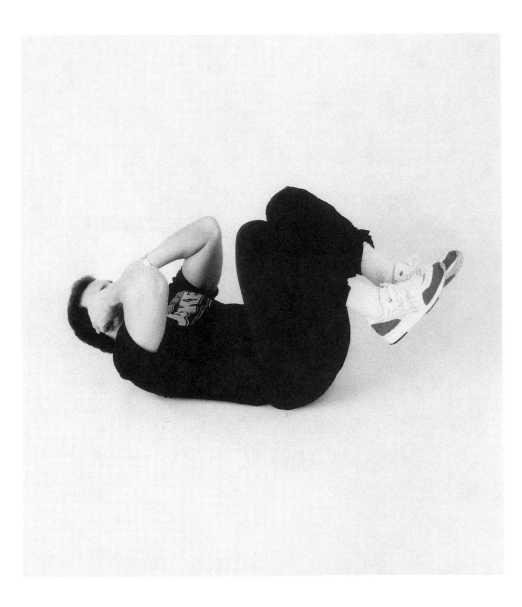

7. KICK-OUT

Place your hands below your buttisimo to support the tailbone. Arms are flexed. Head should be on the ground for beginners and lifted slightly for pros. Breathe out as you kick out, not extending the legs all the way. Great exercise for lower stomach and upper thighs.

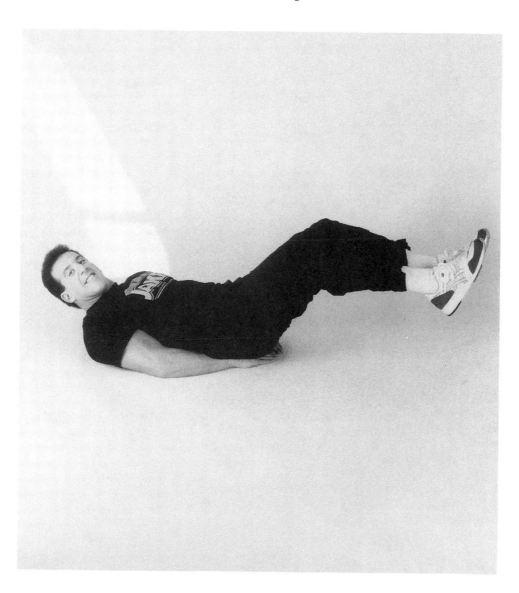

8. SKY HIGH

Begin with your knees bent and feet flat on the ground. With your palms facing each other and your arms extended to the ceiling, breathe out as you reach up. Be sure and squeeze that buttisimo and keep your back flat on the ground. Make sure you raise your shoulders off the ground and keep your back flat.

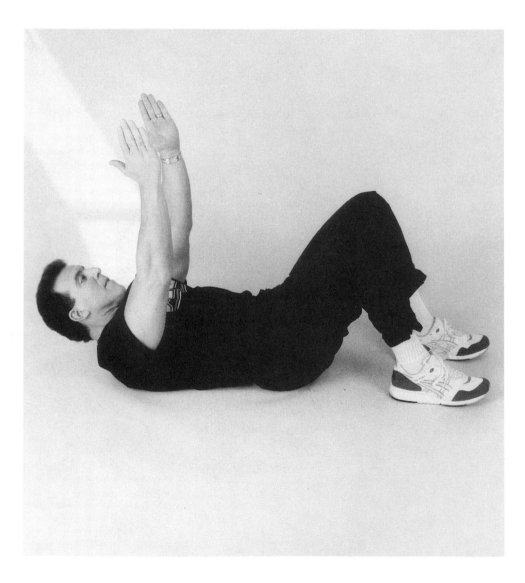

9. BICEP CURL

Start in the Jake stance with a pair of weights and your arms shoulder-width apart. Lift weights to shoulder height and then extend your arms back down. Feel the resistance on the way up and on the way down. Make sure not to lock out the elbows at any time.

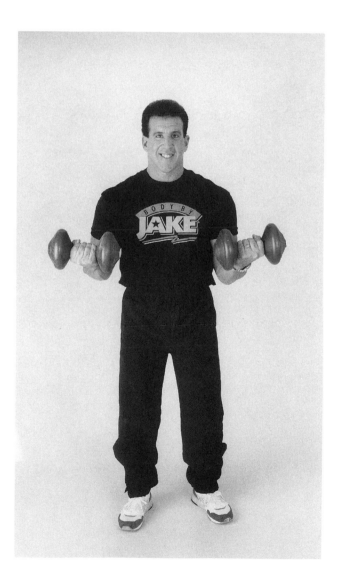

10. TRICEP KICK-OUT

Grab your weights. Stand with your feet shoulder-width apart and your knees slightly bent. Bend over slightly but keep your back flat and kick out behind you with your arms. Bring back to starting position. Keep the whole body tight. Make sure your body is at a forty-five degree angle, elbows close to your sides. Kick the weights out and bring back slowly. Don't swing your arms.

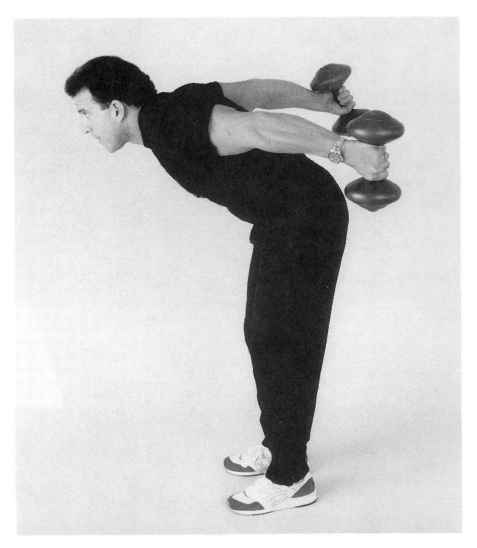

SUCCESS TIPS

The hardest part of exercising might be motivating yourself to do it three to five times a week. Like anything else, there are factors under your control that will help you get (and keep) going.

1. *Schedule* your exercise like any other "appointment." When was the last time you said, "Gee, I have nothing to do for the next hour?" When was the last time that happened five times in a week? Exercise can become a habit if you "ink it in" and then just follow through.

2. Make sure you set *reasonable goals.* Chances are running ten miles a day isn't realistic. Neither is exercising seven days a week. The more realistic your goals, the easier it will be to fulfill them.

3. Start *slowly* if you haven't exercised for a while. Expect to experience a little muscle soreness and stiffness for the first few days. That will go away soon. If you don't try to do too much too fast, you'll make steady progress toward a healthier, leaner you. And most of all, you won't quit.

4. Ask *friends* to exercise with you. You'll encourage and motivate each other. You'll have someone to talk to. You'll find the time passes more quickly.

5. Think about the *location* where you are exercising. The middle of the family room floor, with the dog licking your face, is not the spot! Find an out-of-the-way but comfortable spot where distractions are minimized. If you are working out at a club, find one where most members are "like you." If you're just starting, you may find the less Lycra and tank tops the better.

6. Exercise the same *time* each day. This helps you integrate your workout into your schedule more easily. Soon, it will seem like just another "normal" part of your day.

7. Remember that *participation* not perfection is the goal of exercise. If you miss a workout or just can't get going one day, so what! Don't get hung up on it. Just get back on track the next day.

8. Keep *variety* in your program to fight boredom. I've included many different routines in my exercise program to show you just how varied a program can be and still be effective. If you are tired of one exercise, try another.

9. *Distract* yourself if you find it helps. With an inexpensive tape player or radio on your hip, you can learn a new language, listen to your favorite music or catch up on the news. This is a super-productive thirty minutes for your brain and body!

10. Remind yourself how *good* you feel after you exercise. That great, alive, "with it" feeling is your reward for doing something good for yourself. Remember, you only get it...if you do it!

AND KEEP IN MIND

You may already be doing more exercise than you realize. Many of the sports we enjoy most are terrific forms of exercise. Or if you live in a house with lots of stairs, you may be getting a great daily workout.

To enhance the benefits derived from some common forms of exercise, here are some tips worth keeping in mind.

AEROBIC DANCE

Tip

Find an instructor you like who goes at a pace that is comfortable for you. Wear good shoes. Get into a three-days-a-week routine at a time that will be convenient for you. Have fun, make it social, and encourage your classmates!

Benefit

Excellent for toning and cardiovascular activity.

BICYCLING

Tip

Find a cycling "buddy" to ride with you on weekends (or anytime). Wear a helmet. Keep up a good, steady pace of about eighty pedals a minute.

Benefit

One of the best all-round exercises if you push yourself hard enough. Great for aerobic benefit and weight loss while firming the legs and buttisimo without pounding or jarring.

GOLF

Tip

Walk the course at a nice pace. Try to carry your own bag.

Benefit

Good for eye and hand coordination. Also helps keep the upper body flexible. Walking the course tones the legs and gives the heart some work. The faster you pace yourself, the greater the benefit.

ROWING

Tip

Maintain a smooth, even rhythm. If you're doing your rowing on a machine rather than on a lake, wear lifting gloves if your hands aren't used to the machine. Pretend you are on a college rowing team with others!

Benefit

Tremendous for upper body, leg strength, and heart.

RUNNING

Tip

Get some good shoes that fit properly. Don't be afraid to stop and walk for awhile. If possible, run in dirt or grass rather than on asphalt or concrete. It's easier on the joints.

Benefit

Good cardiovascular exercise. Plus tones legs and helps control weight.

STAIR CLIMBING

Tip

Whether you're climbing stairs at home or at work, or doing your climbing on a machine at the gym, I suggest you monitor your pulse the first few times to find a pace that increases your heart rate. You'll quickly settle into that pace at each workout.

Benefit

Tones legs, thighs, and buttisimo. Good for overall fitness.

SWIMMING

Tip

Try goggles if the chlorine bothers your eyes. Vary your stroke.

Benefit

One of the best all-round exercises. Great for aerobic fitness, arms and shoulders, and flexibility.

TENNIS/RACQUETBALL

Tip

Take some lessons early to help develop a good swing and understanding of the game. Find partners to play with that are at your skill level.

Benefit

Good for agility, hand and eye coordination, and overall toning.

WALKING

Tip

Walk with a partner or partners. To walk more quickly, try pumping your arms harder and faster. Don't be afraid to vary your pace according to your heartbeat and how you feel. Wear comfortable shoes.

Benefit

Consistent walking is a good method of weight control. Promotes toning of the lower body, and if you swing your arms you can get an overall toning effect. Walk fast enough to break a sweat and it's the equivalent of running a nine-minute mile pace (without the jolt).

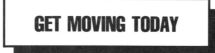

7

JAKE'S BIG TEN: MENTAL EXERCISES

Mental fitness is a state of mind. It's about flexing your willpower, exerting a positive influence on the events in your life, and pulling yourself up to and beyond your own standards of excellence.

Whew!

I break out into a sweat just thinking about mental fitness.

But achieving mental fitness takes as much work and effort as shaping your muscles. It's easy to become lazy about maintaining an upbeat attitude.

So how do you become mentally fit? Here are some of the favorite mind "exercises" that I've used over the years.

1. THE S-T-R-E-T-C-H

Always reach for more than you think you can accomplish. If your goal is to open your own retail store, aim higher and create your own chain. If you're trying to break into acting, push yourself to win an Oscar. You know what? You might surprise yourself one day!

2. THE JAKE JUGGLE

Keep several balls in the air at the same time. In other words, always have several projects going at once. This way, if one or two don't succeed, you've still got other things going.

3. THE SPRINT

Act quickly when opportunity knocks. Windows of opportunity have a way of closing quickly. It's better to be a day early than a minute late. Speed is an essential ingredient in success. If somebody offers you a good price for a home you're selling, respond quickly or you could lose the sale. If you hear of an attractive job opening, call immediately. When somebody asks for something in a week, I always try to get it to them tomorrow.

4. THE FULL-COURT PRESS

Pursue your top goals and fulfill your most important responsibilities with complete dedication and energy. These parts of your life demand your *full* attention. Don't be carefree about the important goals and responsibilities in your life. Let's say you're interviewing for a new job. Find out everything you can about the company and its competitors. Solicit advice from business associates. Write a follow-up letter to the people who interviewed you, thanking them for their time.

5. THE CHIN-UP

Carry yourself with an air of quiet confidence, control, and dignity. If you project these qualities, it will be easy for others to believe in you and have confidence in your abilities.

6. SHADOW BOXING

Work out your frustrations on imaginary targets. If your job's got you down, go for a vigorous run. If the kids are driving you crazy, throw a ball against the wall for a few minutes. Take a walk. Play a game of tennis. The point is to release pent-up feelings harmlessly through physical activity. You'll be surprised how much better it makes you feel.

7. THE SWAN DIVE

Push yourself to plunge headfirst into new experiences. Approach these new experiences with vigor and enthusiasm whether they relate to your personal or professional life. Make a splash! My first body-building competition was a nerve-wracking experience. I could have flopped badly. But I forced myself to overcome my inexperience by throwing myself into the heat of the competition. And I took home a trophy.

8. THE HIGH HURDLE

Challenges in life are not necessarily insurmountable brick walls. Think of them as a series of hurdles. Vault them with a combination of power, grace, and timing.

9. THE HIGH-WIRE BALANCING ACT

Sometimes you'll find yourself walking a tightrope...without a net! For example, you're suddenly called on to make a speech. Or you agree to take on an additional assignment at work, though you're swamped by your current load. Treat these moments as unique opportunities. You'll find that you probably have a tremendous capacity not only to survive these "dangerous" moments but to succeed as well. Remember, walking the tightrope gives you a chance to shine in the spotlight.

10. THE MARATHON

Remember that life is not a sprint, it's a marathon. Don't be discouraged by short-term setbacks or disappointments. Keep your eye on the big picture and accomplishment of the long-term goal. And most of all, enjoy the scenery along the way. That's the way to cross the finish line a winner!

DON'T QUIT!

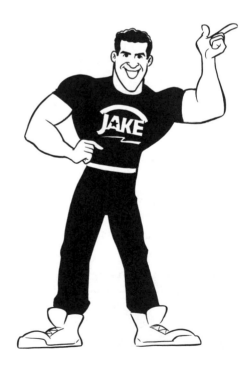

YOU ARE WHAT YOU EAT

Let's face it. You ARE what you EAT and there's no getting around it. If your diet consists primarily of ice cream and donuts, you're not going to have the energy and stamina it takes to make it a winning day. Eat foods that give you high energy and that don't slow you down in the long run. It's really that simple.

It's easy to get confused about what to eat in order to stay healthy and trim. To help myself and others, I devised a nutrition plan called the "Ten in 21" program. Basically, it's about losing ten pounds in twenty-one days without the use of powders, pills, or seaweed. It's a lifestyle program. To go into all of its components would take a whole other book, but what I've done here is to distill some of the most important elements from that program—those guaranteed to bring out the winner in you.

1. CALORIES COUNT

As a rule, if you are moderately active, multiply your *desired* (not actual) weight by twelve to determine how many calories you need a day. If you are relatively inactive, multiply by ten. If you are very active, multiply by fourteen.

2. DON'T BE IN THE DARK ABOUT THE COLOR OF FOOD

For the most part, the deeper the color of fruits and vegetables, the more nutrients they contain. For example, light green iceberg lettuce has only nineteen grams of calcium, whereas the dark romaine lettuce contains sixty-eight grams.

3. FIVE A DAY

Eat five servings of fruits and vegetable (combined) a day. Remember, *raw* vegetables and fresh fruits have the most nutrients. So, do as I do, and try to have a bowl of seasonal fruits always nearby, and some cut up vegetables handy in the refrigerator.

4. SOFT EQUALS LESS FAT

Generally, the softer the margarine, the less saturated it is. The less saturated the fat, the better off you'll be. Tub margarines are usually better than soft sticks because they contain more air and water.

5. WHAT'S YOUR BEEF?

When choosing hamburger, look for meat that has a medium-to-deep color indicating it has a lower fat content, or buy meat labeled "extra lean."

6. READ THE FINE PRINT

Be sure to check the ingredient labels on all food packages. The first ingredient of the label is the one with the highest content. Your margarine at home should have a liquid vegetable oil first on the label rather than a "partially hydrogenated" oil.

7. EASY ON THE SPREAD

Keep butter or margarine at room temperature. It not only makes it easier to spread on your bread, but you'll probably spread less of it than when it's cold. And that means you'll be eating less fat and calories. If you're willing to forgo butter or margarine on your bread altogether, try pureeing your favorite fruits and using them as spreads instead.

8. THE COLD FACTS ABOUT FAT

Refrigerate canned stews, soups, gravies, and other canned foods. The fat will collect and rise to the top, which makes it easy to scrape off.

9. COUNT FAT CALORIES

How do you determine the percentage of fat in packaged foods? Try using this formula:

$$\frac{(\text{Grams of fat per serving}) \times 9}{\text{Total calories per serving}}$$

So if you ate a 130-calorie single serving of packaged food that had four grams of fat, it would be 28 percent fat.

1. (4 grams of fat) $\times$ 9 = 36
2. 36/130 = 28 percent fat

10. SKIM IT DOWN

Switching from whole to skim milk saves you a lot of fat calories, but if you try to make the change all at once, skim can taste pretty bland. Try this: start by mixing half whole milk and half 2 percent milk. After a week or so, try 2 percent mixed with 1 percent and so on. Eventually skim milk will taste normal. Your bones (and heart!) will love you for it.

11. CARBO STARTERS

Starting meals with a high-carbohydrate food like a pasta appetizer or bread without butter actually lessens your fat craving as the meal continues. This way, you won't be as likely to want a high-fat dessert.

12. THE STICKING POINT

Cook with nonstick pots and pans so you won't have to add as much oil. Or use a nonstick, nonfat cooking spray.

13. DIRTY YOLKS

Here's a neat idea. Try making your omelets with three egg whites but only two egg yolks. You'll cut a third of the cholesterol and never notice the difference. (Don't be afraid to ask them to do this at a restaurant either—any cook worth his "salt" can separate whites and yolks.) You can also mix half whole eggs with half egg substitute.

14. HAVE YOUR STEAK AND EAT IT TOO!

Avoid fatty cuts of steak like New York Strip or Delmonico. Instead, try flank steak, which is leaner. Broil it, then be sure to slice it across the grain. You'll get a nice tender meat with a lot less fat.

15. CHEZ HEALTH

Be a healthy cook! Trim fat from meat and remove skin from poultry before cooking. Experiment with spices instead of salt to add flavor to low-fat dishes. Extracts such as vanilla, almond, peppermint, and orange can add sweetness without sugar.

16. HOME SWEET HOME

It's healthier eating breakfast at home. A Kent State study found that a breakfast eaten at home averages only about 27 percent of its calories from fat, while those eaten out average 35 percent.

17. SLOW DOWN BEFORE IT GOES DOWN

Chew your food slowly. Savor it. Put your utensils down between bites. You'll probably eat less food this way and enjoy it more. I also suggest making mealtime a social time. If you're involved in good conversation, you're less likely to eat too much too quickly.

18. DON'T LET THE LABEL FOOL YOU!

"Light" doesn't necessarily mean low in calories. It could mean light in color or weight consistency. "Light" may also mean that it's lighter than it was before, but it may still not be healthy to eat. Train yourself to look beyond the name and look into the ingredients listed on the package.

19. FOOD ISN'T ALWAYS THE ANSWER

Feeling blue, bored, or under the weather? Think about what you can do *instead* of eating. Take a walk, go for a swim, do a little gardening, pick up the phone and call a friend, take a long, luxurious bath—but stay away from the kitchen.

20. THINK AHEAD

If you can, fix meals ahead of time when you're *not* hungry. Prepare only what you'll eat, or package up the rest immediately and get it into that freezer!

21. WATCH YOUR LANGUAGE

Look for certain foreign cooking terms that figuratively translate to "fat added." *Sauté* means "butter sauce." *Tempura* means "fried in batter." *Au gratin* indicates that the dish has cheese sauce. *Broiling* sounds perfectly safe, and it is...unless it's broiled with butter. Don't hesitate to ask your waiter how the food will be prepared.

Of course, these twenty-one health tips don't cover everything, but they will help you focus on some pretty major areas like cutting fat from your diet and increasing your energy level. Just remember, when it comes to nutrition, *keep it simple.*

IN A NUTSHELL:
Avoid fat as much as possible, and eat plenty of foods high in carbohydrates, nutrients, and vitamins. The lower your intake of fat, the higher your level of energy, and the better your chances are to making it a WINNING DAY!

EAT FIT · DON'T QUIT!

SETBACKS

If you're reading this chapter, it probably means that things aren't going as well as you had planned. Maybe you feel like you're in a slump, and you just can't seem to get yourself out of it. Maybe things just aren't going the way you want them to.

Well, believe me, I know how you're feeling. But as bad as things may seem, you can still reach your goal. I know how unbelievable that can sound to you. But it's absolutely true. As it says in the "Don't Quit" poem:

"IT'S WHEN THINGS SEEM WORST THAT YOU MUST NOT QUIT."

Keep in mind that, when I refer to setbacks, I'm not talking about tragedies. A setback is an unpleasant occurrence, a bit of bad news, or an unwanted dose of the unexpected. For instance:

Your proposal was rejected at work.
You find out your child needs braces . . . and you can't afford them.
You missed an important meeting.
Your car needs a new transmission.
You got passed over for a promotion.
Your dinner flopped.
You ate the double chocolate cake and went off your diet.

The important thing to remember is that it's not the end of the world. It's a setback, sure. But that's all it is. You've been knocked off course slightly. And maybe that makes you feel angry or upset. You don't have to bury those emotions, which are only natural to feel. But you've got to:

■ Analyze what went wrong.
■ Put it in the proper perspective.
■ Learn to channel all your emotions into a positive course to get you back on track.
■ Remember that it's only a temporary obstacle and that you *will* overcome it.

MY SETBACK STORY

In the mid-1980s, I was fortunate to land a part in an ABC sitcom "Shaping Up," with Leslie Nielsen. It was a short-lived comedy set in a health club. I got a role as an airline attendant who was a fitness buff. As proud as I was to get a part in a network program, I was extremely sensitive to being typecast as a musclehead.

Everyone on the show told me I was funny. However, when the first major review came out, it read, "Jake Steinfeld, as the gym *dumbbell*. . . ."

I turned pale. It was exactly what I *didn't* want written about me. I thought I would be washed out of the business.

I immediately turned to several friends for advice, including Harrison Ford. "Hey man, at least they're writing about you," he laughed. "And don't worry about it. It happens to everyone." Three days later, NBC called for me to read for another role as a lady's man. And you know what? I got that part.

My setback is a good example because we're always getting "reviewed" in our lives. It might be a corporate salary review, a comment from your kids on your parenting style, or a grade from your teacher. Expect to be judged. And expect some of those judgments to be harsh. It can't be avoided.

But you *can* bounce back. That one review rocked me. *It set me back.* It wasn't what I wanted to hear. But I never gave up. It didn't stop me from trying again and again. It became a learning experience. And this is what I learned from that one small incident about how to deal with a setback.

EVERYONE VISITS SETBACK CITY

It's not a spot on any map, but you know the place. It's where a dream slipped away. Or a junction in the road where a smooth journey turned into a rough ride. You hoped to hear yes. You got no. You wanted good news. You got bad. You wanted to do *X*. But instead you did *Y.*

The point is this: We've all been there. That's right. Me. You. Everyone. Anyone can have a setback. And everyone does. Presidents don't win every battle with Congress. Executives don't make every deal. Singers don't hit every note. The best hitters in baseball strike out.

From personal experience, I know that even some of the most glamorous Hollywood stars I've trained over the years have sometimes felt like nothing was going their way. But they overcame these feelings and became successful for two reasons:

1. They learned how to deal with the inevitable setbacks and bounce back.

2. They didn't quit.

Try to accept the universality of setbacks—that they happen to everyone. That recognition becomes a healthy foundation for dealing with them.

Sure, setbacks are tough to take. And it's okay to feel irritated or even down. But you've got to move quickly beyond these feelings. Once you accept that *everyone* has setbacks, you will get back on a more positive track. And most of all, never, ever *QUIT*!

FIND THE POSITIVE SIDE OF A SETBACK

Failure means you tried. And that's good.

> ## YOU CAN'T WIN IF YOU DON'T PLAY.

As I mentioned earlier, when I was in eighth grade, I didn't make the school basketball team. I was crushed. But not for long. That setback made me a better ball player because I practiced day and night for months. I not only made the freshman team the following year, I became a starter.

All setbacks have the potential to become positive forces in your life. Imagine that you've just learned your child needs glasses. That's not the best news in the world. But at least you now know why your child has been suffering from headaches! And maybe the need for glasses explains the recent drop in your child's grades.

Or maybe you didn't get the promotion or raise you deserved. That can hurt or even make you angry. But use those feelings to try harder or push yourself to rewrite your résumé in a search for a better job.

Look for positive elements in a setback and focus on them.

RESPOND QUICKLY AND POSITIVELY TO A SETBACK

A setback can be a deflating experience. There's almost a knee-jerk reaction to collapse and resign yourself to defeat.

Don't give in to this!

It's at these moments that you must be at your sharpest. Be creative. Be decisive. Be determined.

For instance, if you're having a dinner party and your casserole burns, come out of the kitchen with a smile and say, "Guess what? We're having take-out Chinese tonight."

Or if your idea was rejected at a business meeting, come back immediately with another plan.

Life's too short to make yourself nuts with these annoying curve balls. Instead, turn a setback into a win. You can do it if you remember these points:

- Be flexible.
- Have a backup plan.
- Don't lose your cool.

Following these points will enable you to examine your options calmly and help you respond productively.

REGROUP

A setback is a time to circle the wagons, take stock of yourself, and formulate a new plan of action. This regrouping process can take place quickly in a moment of crisis, or it can occur slowly over a period of many days or even weeks.

REGROUPING IS A DEFENSIVE ACTION.

Regrouping buys you some time. It allows you to gather your thoughts. It prepares you to make your next move a *smart* move. It prevents you from acting before thinking.

TALK IT OUT

Your friends and family will be your strongest allies during a setback. I'm a big fan of communicating with friends and family, and a setback is when you really need them. Go to people who are good listeners, clear thinkers, and naturally upbeat. Look to them for ideas, support, and a different perspective.

MISERY LOVES COMPANY
BUT WINNERS LOOK FOR CONSTRUCTIVE ADVICE.

Confront your setback, but don't wallow in it.

You've got to be honest with yourself. And demand honesty from those around you. It's the only way to turn a setback into a positive learning experience.

WRITE IT DOWN

Setbacks can confuse us. They are things we often try to push out of our minds. But in order to learn from setbacks, it's necessary to confront them. And to do that, it often helps to write yourself a short note about what went wrong. This serves several purposes:

1. It clarifies the event.
2. It forces you to deal with the setback.
3. It helps you find a solution to the setback.
4. It becomes a positive reference tool for dealing with future setbacks.

When I first arrived in Los Angeles, my goal was to win a local body-building competition. I trained a full year. My life was totally focused on entering and winning that competition. Unfortunately, I came in second. What made the loss so difficult was that I suspected the winner used steroids. I realized that the only way I could win in future body-building competition was to take the steroids. (This was, after all, the innocent days of 1979.) That was clearly unacceptable. I was confused, angry, and hurt. I didn't know what to do. One night, I simply sat down and wrote myself this short note:

> I love working out. I love what it does for my body and my mind. I love competing. But I will not use steroids to enhance my physique or to compete in bodybuilding competition. Therefore, it's doubtful I'll be able to compete successfully in professional body-building competitions. I must seek alternative options. I have to open other doors in this field.

That short note sharpened my thinking. It helped put me on the path that I'm on today. I'm glad I saved that note. Today, looking back on it, my dilemma seems trivial.

Keep your notes after your setbacks. They'll help improve your vision as you review your past accomplishments and challenges. I promise you: a few months after you've overcome your setback, you'll read your note and think, "I can't believe I was so upset about *that* incident."

GET BACK IN THE SADDLE

If a horse throws you, what do you do? You get back in the saddle.

Same thing with a setback. If you went off your diet, start dieting again. If the boss didn't like your proposal, come up with another one. If someone turned you down for a date, call up someone else.

But remember—jump into action only when you're ready. Make sure you're confident. Make sure you've analyzed the problem. Make sure you know what your game plan is. Make sure you've formed a positive picture in your head.

Three days after my negative review in the sitcom "Shaping Up," I went right out and auditioned for another role. In those seventy-two hours, I had analyzed what went wrong. I consulted with friends. And I got *way* beyond my initial hurt and disappointment. My confidence was restored, and I was ready to face the outside world once again. And once again, I believed in myself and my abilities.

> # IF YOU BELIEVE IN YOURSELF, OTHERS WILL BELIEVE IN YOU.

It's really that simple.

IN A NUTSHELL, a setback is not the end of the world. It's a *temporary* detour on your road to success.

Setbacks have positive elements. They're growth experiences. They challenge us. They force us to grow closer to friends and family. They help us reexamine our lives and goals.

To deal most productively with a setback, you must:

- Remember that setbacks happen to everyone.
- Respond positively.
- Reflect on what went wrong.
- Seek advice from those closest to you.
- Get back into the game.

Ultimately, there's only one way to think about a setback.

> # A SETBACK IS A LEARNING EXPERIENCE, NOT A FAILURE.

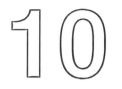

10

THE JAKE CHALLENGE

I've shown you throughout the book how a regular guy like myself can become a winner in body, mind, and spirit. If I can do it, I KNOW you can. Here's my challenge...

- I challenge you to wake up every morning with a smile.

- I challenge you to look yourself in the mirror and be honest.

- I challenge you to never accept the word no.

- I challenge you to discuss your highs and lows with your close friends and family.

- I challenge you to make exercise and nutrition an important part of your life.

- I challenge you to take time for your family and your own personal interests.

- I challenge to go out there and WIN.

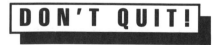

DON'T QUIT!

11

THE "DON'T QUIT" POEM

"DON'T QUIT"

When things go wrong as they sometimes will,
When the road you're trudging seems all uphill,
When the funds are low, and the debts are high,
And you want to smile, but you have to sigh,
When care is pressing you down a bit,
Rest, if you must, but do not quit.

Life is queer, with its twists and turns
As every one of us sometimes learns.
And many a failure turns about
When he might have won had he stuck it out.
Don't give up, though the pace seems slow.
You may succeed with another blow.

Success is failure turned inside out—
The silver tint of the clouds of doubt.
And you never can tell how close you are.
It may be near when it seems so far.
So stick to the fight when you're hardest hit.
It's when things seem worst that you must not quit.

I'd love to hear from you.
If you'd like to be placed
on my mailing list, write to:

Body by Jake
P.O. Box 1800
Spring Valley, CA 91979